# HEALTH CARE IN DIGITAL ERA

## UNDERSTANDING ALL THE TECHNOLOGIES
## FOR HEALTHCARE

## KATE .P

# Contents

# CHAPTER ONE

## Introduction

Healthcare has changed dramatically in the digital age, changing how medical services are handled, accessed, and provided. The purpose of this introduction is to give a general overview of healthcare in the digital age, emphasizing significant developments, difficulties, and possibilities.

1. Technologies for Digital Health:

Artificial intelligence (AI) systems, wearable technology, health applications, electronic health records (EHRs), and telemedicine are just a few examples of the many instruments that fall under the umbrella of digital health technologies. These technologies provide remote health status monitoring, diagnosis, treatment, and management, hence enhancing individualized and effective healthcare delivery.

2. Remote Care and Telemedicine:

With the rise in popularity of telemedicine, patients can now consult with medical professionals at a distance using encrypted messaging apps, phone calls, or video calls. This strategy minimizes the need for in-person visits and lowers healthcare expenditures while improving access to healthcare, especially in rural or underserved areas.

3. Health monitoring and wearable technology:

Vital signs, activity levels, and health data can be continuously monitored with wearable technology, including smartwatches, fitness trackers, and medical sensors. These gadgets give people the confidence to take charge of their health and give medical practitioners useful real-time data for diagnosis and therapy.

4. EHRs, or electronic health records:

Electronic Health Records (EHRs) digitize patient health data, enabling smooth provider collaboration and communication, enhancing care coordination, and lowering medical errors. EHRs facilitate data analytics and research endeavors, providing valuable insights into treatment outcomes and trends in population health.

5. Healthcare and Artificial Intelligence:

Healthcare is undergoing a transformation thanks to artificial intelligence (AI) technologies, such as machine learning and natural language processing, which improve diagnostic accuracy, anticipate illness risk, optimize treatment regimens, and streamline administrative processes. Applications for artificial intelligence (AI) span the gamut, from virtual health assistants and personalized treatment to drug discovery and medical imaging analysis.

6. Security and Privacy of Data:

Patient data security and privacy must be guaranteed as healthcare data becomes more digitally connected and digitalized. To protect sensitive health data, healthcare institutions need to put strong cybersecurity protections in place, follow stringent regulatory standards, and give patient consent and data openness first priority.

7. Difficulties and Ethical Issues:

Healthcare digitization has a number of difficulties, such as unequal digital access, problems with system interoperability, data interoperability, and ethical questions about the use of AI and patient data. To tackle these obstacles, cooperation amongst concerned parties, infrastructure spending, and the creation of all-encompassing legal structures are necessary.

8. Prospective Courses:

Looking ahead, there is a ton of room for innovation and change in the healthcare industry in the digital age. New technologies that are poised to further change personalized medicine, disease prevention, and healthcare delivery include genomics, blockchain, and virtual reality. The future of digital health will be shaped by ongoing investments in worker training, technology adoption, and research.

A new era of healthcare marked by unparalleled connectedness, innovation, and patient-centric care has been brought about by the digital revolution. Healthcare stakeholders may solve current issues, enhance clinical outcomes, and enable people to live healthier lives by utilizing digital technologies.

# The impact of the digital era on healthcare

The advent of digital technology has significantly transformed the healthcare sector in a number of ways.

Improved Access to Care: People, particularly those living in rural or underserved areas, now have easier access to healthcare thanks to telemedicine and smartphone health apps. Through digital platforms, patients may now make appointments, obtain medical information, communicate with healthcare practitioners remotely, and even obtain prescriptions.

Enhanced Patient Involvement: Thanks to digital technologies, patients are now better equipped to actively manage their health. Individuals can monitor chronic diseases, set health goals, measure vital signs, and improve communication with healthcare professionals by using wearable devices, health monitoring applications, and patient portals.

Effective Healthcare Delivery: By digitizing patient health information, electronic health records, or EHRs, have made it possible for healthcare workers to collaborate and communicate more easily. In the end, this has enhanced care coordination, decreased paperwork, minimized errors, and streamlined administrative activities, all of which have contributed to more effective healthcare delivery.

Precision Medicine: This field of medicine, which customizes medical care and preventive measures to individual traits including genetics, lifestyle, and environment, was made possible by advancements in genome sequencing, data analytics, and artificial intelligence. By more precisely targeting interventions, this personalized strategy has the potential to improve patient outcomes and save healthcare expenditures.

Diagnostic Advancements: The accuracy and efficiency of disease detection and diagnosis have been greatly enhanced by AI-powered medical imaging and diagnostic systems. Medical photos, pathology slides, and patient data can all be analyzed by machine learning algorithms to find trends, estimate the risk of disease, and help doctors make decisions.

Innovation in Healthcare: With startups, tech businesses, and research institutes creating ground-breaking technologies and solutions, the digital age has sparked innovation in the healthcare sector. These breakthroughs, which range from blockchain for safe health data exchange to virtual reality for pain management, have the potential to revolutionize healthcare delivery, enhance patient outcomes, and reduce costs.

Data-driven Insights: Patient records, clinical trial data, and population health data are just a few examples of the vast amounts of health data that big data analytics allow healthcare businesses to extract insights from. These insights have the potential to improve resource allocation, forecast disease outbreaks, spot trends and patterns, and influence healthcare policy—all of which can result in more successful public health initiatives and healthcare interventions.

Problems and Considerations: Although the digital transformation of healthcare has many advantages, there are drawbacks as well. These include worries about data security and privacy, problems with interoperability between various systems, unequal access to digital resources, and ethical issues with the use of AI and machine learning in healthcare decision-making. Collaboration across stakeholders, strong regulatory frameworks, and continuous innovation in technology and healthcare delivery models are necessary to meet these issues.

The digital age has completely changed the healthcare industry, presenting previously unheard-of chances to boost productivity, spur innovation, and improve patient care. Healthcare stakeholders can solve present issues and clear the path for a healthier, more connected future by ethically and inclusively utilizing the power of digital technologies.

## Telemedicine

The term "telemedicine" describes the use of telecommunications technology to provide medical treatments remotely. It includes a wide range of services that are delivered remotely via phone calls, secure messaging apps, video calls, and other digital communication devices. These services include consultations, diagnosis, monitoring, and treatment.

**Important telemedicine features include:**

Remote Consultations: Patients can have consultations with medical professionals via telemedicine from the comfort of their homes or other convenient locations. Without the need for in-person visits, patients can discuss their symptoms, get advice from medical professionals, and even get prescriptions filled through video conversations or encrypted messaging platforms.

# CHAPTER TWO

Access to Specialists: By linking patients with specialists who might not be available locally, telemedicine helps patients get past geographic obstacles. People who live in underserved or rural locations, where access to specialty care may be limited, will especially benefit from this.

Chronic Disease Management: By enabling remote monitoring and follow-up care, telemedicine helps with the continuous management of chronic illnesses. Wearable technology and health monitoring apps allow patients with illnesses like diabetes, hypertension, or heart disease to keep track of their health metrics and exchange information with their healthcare providers for prompt intervention and treatment plan modifications.

Emergency Care & Triage: By offering remote triage and preliminary assessments, telemedicine can be extremely helpful in emergency situations. Telemedicine can assist in assessing the severity of an emergency, offering advice on first aid procedures, and expediting the dispatch of emergency services when prompt medical assistance is needed.

Telepsychiatry and Mental Health Services: The provision of mental health services, such as counseling, therapy, and psychiatric consultations, has shown to be very successful when carried out using telemedicine. Video-based sessions lessen stigma and improve access to care for those in need by enabling people to get mental health help in the comfort of their own homes.

Follow-up Care and Postoperative Monitoring: By allowing medical professionals to consult with patients following surgeries or hospital stays, telemedicine helps to minimize the need for pointless clinic visits and lowers the possibility of problems. Patients can communicate remotely about their progress, voice any worries, and get advice on aftercare.

Time and Money Savings: Telemedicine helps patients and healthcare professionals save money and time. Healthcare providers can streamline their schedules and cut costs associated with operating physical clinics, while patients can avoid travel fees and time away from work or other commitments associated with in-person consultations.

Telemedicine has many advantages, but it also has drawbacks, such as difficulties with reimbursement, technological constraints, privacy and security of patient data, and legal obstacles. To address these issues and guarantee the efficient and secure provision of telemedicine services, thorough legislative frameworks must be developed, infrastructure and technological investments must be made, and stakeholder participation is essential.

All things considered, telemedicine has great potential to increase patient outcomes, increase access to care, and improve the effectiveness of healthcare delivery especially in the digital age when connectivity and remote communication are becoming more and more common.

## Applications for Health

Apps that support and encourage different facets of health and wellness are referred to as health apps, or mobile health (mHealth) apps. These apps, which range in functionality from mental health support and chronic disease management to fitness tracking and nutrition management, are usually accessible for download on smartphones and tablets. An outline of health apps' salient characteristics is provided below:

Fitness and Activity Tracking: Personal trainers, workout logs, and fitness objectives can all be managed with the use of fitness applications. They frequently interface with wearable technology, such as smartwatches or fitness trackers, to gather information on steps taken, distance traveled, calories burned, and heart rate. To assist users in staying motivated and reaching their fitness goals, several applications also include capabilities for tracking progress, demonstrations of exercises, and customized training routines.

Nutrition and Diet Management: Users can count calories, keep an eye on their eating patterns, and choose healthier foods with the help of nutrition applications. Features like meal planning, barcode scanning for nutritional data, recipe libraries, food journaling, and personalized nutrition recommendations based on dietary choices or personal health objectives are a few examples of what these applications might offer. Additionally, several apps offer features for monitoring the consumption of micronutrients, macronutrient ratios, and water.

Mental Health and Well-Being: Apps for mental health provide tools and assistance in the management of stress, anxiety, depression, and other mental illnesses. Some of the elements that they might offer are guided meditation and mindfulness exercises, mood monitoring, cognitive behavioral therapy (CBT) methods, relaxation techniques, and connections to peer support groups or mental health specialists. These applications seek to enhance coping mechanisms, foster emotional stability, and offer self-care techniques for enhanced mental well-being.

Sleep Tracking and Enhancement: Apps for tracking sleep assist users in keeping an eye on their sleeping habits, evaluating the quality of their sleep, and pinpointing potential sleep-influencing variables. In order to improve sleep patterns, they could include features like smart alarms, bedtime reminders, sleep stage analysis, sleep monitoring algorithms, and sleep hygiene advice. To aid users in de-stressing and facilitating a more effortless sleep, certain applications provide guided nighttime routines, white noise or natural sound effects, and relaxation techniques.

Chronic Disease Management: People who are in charge of long-term medical disorders like diabetes, high blood pressure, asthma, and heart disease can benefit from using health applications. With the help of these apps, users may keep tabs on vital signs, manage symptoms, document medication adherence, and record pertinent health metrics. In order to improve illness management and treatment outcomes, they might also include instructional materials, medication reminders, individualized health insights, and communication channels for data exchange with healthcare practitioners.

Pregnancy tracking and women's health: Applications for women's health address particular issues with menstruation hygiene, fertility monitoring, pregnancy tracking, and reproductive health. Menstrual cycle tracking, ovulation prediction, techniques for fertility awareness, pregnancy tracking tools, information on prenatal care, and postpartum support are just a few of the things they provide. With the help of these applications, women can take charge of their reproductive health and make knowledgeable decisions regarding prenatal care and family planning.

Accessibility and Inclusivity: In order to make sure that people with a range of needs and abilities can use health apps, accessibility and inclusivity are receiving more and more attention. In order to meet the particular health concerns of various communities, this includes elements like customized interfaces, language options, accessibility settings for people with disabilities, and culturally sensitive material.

Even though there are many advantages to using health apps to promote fitness and health, it's important to take into account aspects like app trustworthiness, data privacy, and security while selecting and utilizing these apps. In addition to reading user reviews and ratings and comprehending the app's privacy policies on data collecting, storage, and sharing methods, users should choose reliable apps from reliable developers. Users can also make well-informed judgments about integrating health applications into their daily routine and lifestyle by speaking with trained experts or healthcare professionals.

Electronic health records, or EHRs, are digital copies of paper patient charts that include detailed health information about a patient's medical history, diagnosis, prescriptions, plans of care, dates of immunizations, allergies, results of laboratory tests, radiological pictures, and other pertinent medical data. EHRs are made to be available to authorized healthcare professionals and personnel in a variety of healthcare environments, enabling effective and well-coordinated patient care.

Prominent attributes and advantages of Electronic Health Records (EHRs) encompass:

Centralized Patient Data: By combining patient health data from multiple sources into a single electronic record, electronic health records (EHRs) give medical professionals a thorough understanding of a patient's past medical history and present state of health. By reducing errors and omissions, this centralized information optimizes patient safety, decreases redundant testing, and improves clinical decision-making.

Accessibility and Interoperability: Electronic Health Records (EHRs) allow authorized healthcare providers to safely access patient records from various locations, promoting easy communication and teamwork among members of the care team. In order to guarantee continuity of care and information sharing throughout the healthcare ecosystem, interoperability standards enable EHR systems to communicate data with other healthcare systems and other stakeholders, such as laboratories, pharmacies, and public health organizations.

Clinical Documentation: By allowing healthcare clinicians to electronically record patient interactions, including notes, diagnoses, procedures, and treatment plans, EHRs simplify the processes involved in clinical documentation. In order to assure compliance with regulatory standards, standardize documentation methods, and increase accuracy, templates and organized data entry fields are helpful. Furthermore, more effective documentation procedures are made possible by voice recognition and natural language processing technologies, which lessen administrative load and free up time for patient care.

Clinical decision support technologies, like alerts, reminders, and clinical guidelines, are integrated into electronic health records (EHRs) to help healthcare providers make evidence-based decisions at the point of care. By identifying possible drug interactions, allergy alerts, suggestions for preventive care, and best practices for managing particular medical problems, these technologies can improve patient safety and care quality.

Patient Empowerment and Engagement: By giving patients access to their electronic health records via patient portals or personal health records (PHRs), electronic health records (EHRs) enable people to take an active role in their healthcare. In order to improve their understanding of their health issues, communicate with their healthcare providers, and participate in shared decision-making regarding their care, patients can access their medical data, lab results, medication lists, appointment schedules, and educational materials.

Quality Improvement and Population Health Management: By gathering and evaluating data on patient demographics, healthcare outcomes, and clinical performance indicators, EHRs assist with both population health management and quality improvement projects. Healthcare organizations can use data analytics technologies to assess performance metrics, spot treatment gaps, keep an eye on population health trends, and launch focused interventions that will enhance patient outcomes and healthcare delivery.

Data Security and Privacy: Electronic Health Records (EHRs) are equipped with strong security features that guard patient health data against cyber threats, illegal access, and breaches. The confidentiality, integrity, and accessibility of electronic health records are protected by encryption, authentication controls, audit trails, and role-based access permissions. These measures also assist ensure compliance with privacy laws like the Health Insurance Portability and Accountability Act (HIPAA).

EHRs have a lot to offer in terms of bettering patient care, productivity, and data management, but they also have drawbacks, including problems with user interface design, a lot of data entry, obstacles to interoperability, and worries about data security and privacy. Investing in technology, staff training, usability testing, and regulatory compliance are necessary to overcome these obstacles and maximize the usage and influence of electronic health records in contemporary healthcare delivery.

In the current healthcare environment, wearable technology and remote monitoring play a vital role by providing creative ways to track health indicators, keep an eye on chronic illnesses, and encourage wellness. An outline of wearable technology and its uses in remote monitoring is provided below:

1. Wearable Technology:

Fitness trackers are wearable gadgets with sensors that measure physical activity parameters like heart rate, steps done, distance traveled, and calories burned. They frequently connect to computer programs or smartphone apps to give users real-time feedback on their workout routines and advancement toward fitness objectives.

Smartwatches: In addition to fitness tracking features, smartwatches are equipped with GPS tracking, heart rate monitoring, sleep tracking, and calendar alerts and call and message notifications. Users can access a variety of health-related features and services by using smartwatches that support third-party health and wellness apps.

Medical wearables: These devices are intended to be used in the management of chronic conditions or the monitoring of particular health metrics. Smart inhalers for managing asthma, wearable ECG monitors for heart rhythm monitoring, and continuous glucose monitors (CGMs) for diabetes management are a few examples. These gadgets assist medical professionals in remotely tracking patient data and give individuals useful insights into their current health.

Wearable Biosensors: These biosensors can measure a range of physiological characteristics, including electrodermal activity, oxygen saturation, body temperature, and respiration rate. They can also measure levels of hydration. They provide continuous vital sign monitoring and early identification of anomalies in health and can be incorporated into apparel, patches, or accessories.

# CHAPTER THREE

2. Applications for Remote Monitoring:

Chronic Illness Management: In order to effectively treat long-term illnesses like diabetes, hypertension, heart disease, and respiratory problems, wearable technology and remote monitoring are essential. Wearable technology enables patients to monitor key health indicators, get immediate feedback on their health, and share information with medical professionals for remote monitoring and treatment.

Postoperative Care: Remote monitoring technologies help with postoperative care by giving medical professionals the ability to keep tabs on patients' vital signs, monitor their state of recovery, and spot any difficulties or unfavorable events. This can ease patient discomfort, lessen the need for in-person clinic visits, and enable early response in the event of a medical emergency.

Aging in Place: With the use of wearable technology and remote monitoring tools, senior citizens can live independently as they age while getting proactive health support and monitoring. Wearable technology and home monitoring systems can incorporate sensors to detect falls, track users' activity levels, remind users to take their medications, and notify emergency services or caregivers in the event of an emergency.

Wellness and Preventive Health: By motivating users to embrace good habits like consistent exercise, a balanced diet, enough sleep, and stress reduction, wearable technology helps users achieve wellness and preventive health. Users may establish and meet health goals, stay motivated, and adopt healthier lifestyles with the support of features like personalized feedback and coaching.

Research & Clinical Trials: Wearables and remote monitoring technologies are being used more often in research studies and clinical trials to gather empirical data on patient outcomes, adherence to treatment plans, and reaction to interventions. These technologies improve the accuracy and dependability of research findings, facilitate remote data collecting, and lessen the workload for study participants.

All things considered, wearable technology and remote monitoring tools are useful resources for encouraging proactive health management, enhancing patient outcomes, and changing the way healthcare is delivered so that it is more patient-centered and data-driven. The uses and effects of remote monitoring in healthcare will grow as long as wearables, data analytics, and networking continue to innovate.

## Summary

In conclusion, a new era of creativity, efficiency, and patient-centricity has been brought about by the merging of digital technologies with healthcare. The digital revolution in healthcare is changing the way medical services are managed, accessed, and delivered. Examples of these innovations include wearable technology, telemedicine, electronic health records (EHRs), and remote monitoring.

Digital health technology have many advantages, such as increased patient engagement, easier access to care, more efficient clinical operations, and improved health outcomes. Data-driven decision-making is supported, communication between healthcare practitioners is facilitated, and patient information is centrally stored in electronic health records. Especially in underprivileged areas, telemedicine enhances care coordination, increases access to healthcare services, and permits remote consultations. People may monitor chronic diseases, take charge of their health, and make educated decisions about their well-being thanks to wearable technology and remote monitoring tools.

There are still obstacles in the way of these developments, such as worries about data security and privacy, interoperability problems, legal restrictions, and unequal access to digital resources. Stakeholder cooperation, technological and infrastructure investments, and the creation of thorough regulatory frameworks to guarantee the secure and efficient application of digital health solutions are all necessary to meet these issues.

Going forward, the digital age in healthcare presents a plethora of opportunities for additional innovation and change. New technologies that have the potential to change healthcare delivery, customized medicine, and population health management include blockchain, virtual reality, genetics, and artificial intelligence. Stakeholders in the healthcare industry may overcome present obstacles, promote good change, and build a future where everyone has access to high-quality, affordable healthcare by responsibly and inclusively utilizing digital technologies.

**THE END**